MINDFUL INTENTIONS

A Personal Guided Journal for Coping with Chronic Pain

Janine Wilburn

WEST
MARGIN
PRESS

I am the day transforming into night

Not quite sure where I am at times

I want to be who I truly am

Not who people always want to be

*I used to be someone who put everything
on my shoulders*

*I have forgotten my hardships,
but I know they have happened*

I hope one day I can just be me

Not be ashamed of it

*I am water crashing up against the rocks,
always hitting, never hurt*

I remember my victories

I let go of my self-doubts

I am life in myself

I am light in others

I want to be everything I am

—C. Wilburn

This journal belongs to

_____

Contents

*Hope is the thing with feathers
That perches in the soul,
And sings the tune
without the words,
And never stops at all...*
—Emily Dickinson

Introduction

Welcome to *Mindful Intentions*! This guided resilience journal is designed with care and based on scientific research, as well as decades of personal experience, to address the unique needs of people living with chronic pain. This book is about enjoying yourself while engaging in entertaining, inspiring, creative, and often pain-reducing activities that are the underpinnings of resilience.

Neuroscience has brought learned people from many disciplines together to study and attempt to understand resiliency. In the study of the brain's neuroplasticity, it is common to see what has once been seen as "softer" or spiritual principles connected to science, and science in turn tracking and explaining the changes in the brain and body based on changes of thought. New discoveries reveal the brain is more malleable than previously understood, and even subtle changes can create new neuropathways that assist in building resilience. The research further reveals that resilience is a skill developed on the physical, emotional, and mental levels—each one interlinked with the other.

Studies continue to focus on how different thought patterns affect the human mind and body. Thoughts trigger cortisol, dopamine, and other hormones and neurotransmitters, which then impact the health and well-being of the body. Some studies suggest that even genes can be positively or negatively affected by our thoughts. Many scientists agree that through choosing specific thought patterns, behaviors, and physical activity, we can become more resilient. For those living in chronic pain, the value of resiliency lies both in the ability to survive what would seem to be devastating experiences, and the ability to move through the challenges of daily life.

This journal contains a number of different types of activities, all designed to work together over time. Every page contains building blocks of resiliency, such as positive writing prompts, inspirational quotes, and fun exercises. You will be guided to create, think positively, be grateful, let go through forgiveness, appreciate what others have done for you, acknowledge your service to others, and more—all actions which are proven to increase resiliency.

By choosing specific thought patterns, behaviors, and physical activities, adults and children can become more resilient—which is exceedingly helpful in dealing with chronic conditions. Equally significant is that the neuroplasticity of the brain allows the brain to continue to change and create new pathways throughout our lives. Therefore, developing regular, ideally daily, practices in any of these areas will help create new neuropathways, bolstering resilience and well-being.

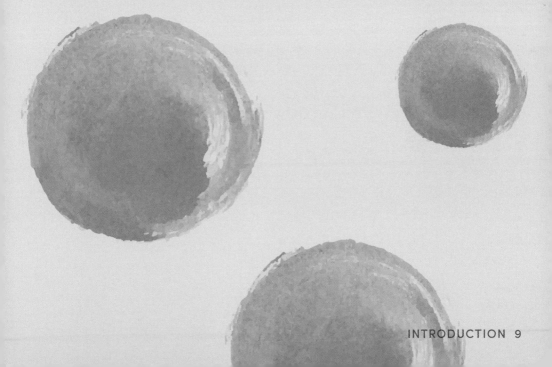

Why I Created This Journal

Resiliency plays a critical role in my daily life, and in my family's life. Twenty-four years ago, I was in a serious car accident. I experienced severe spinal injuries and was given a grim prognosis. This is when I first encountered this distinction in neuroscience called neuroplasticity, through Sharon Begley's book *Train Your Mind, Change Your Brain* and her exploration of Dr. Richard Davidson's research at the University of Wisconsin-Madison (my alma mater). I read and reread the book, and then studied everything I could find on the subject. I knew there were answers in the science to help me heal when most of my doctors and health care practitioners no longer believed it was possible.

I began to engage and develop daily practices that eventually were identified through research as the building blocks of resiliency. The results were overwhelmingly positive. My pain started to diminish and sleep was available for a few hours at a time. I discovered that by being creative I could significantly minimize my pain, so I became a visual artist, even though I had limited use of my hands and arms at the time.

I dug deeper into observing, monitoring, and utilizing my thoughts to enhance my healing, and combined that knowledge and intention to create my many daily practices. In pursuit of a "cure," I found so much more. I learned the importance of love when dealing with hardship. I learned love comes in so many shapes and sizes: forgiveness, gratitude, kindness, creativity, acts of service, authentic listening, compassion, daily practices, prayer, meditation, yoga, still and quiet moments, exercise, and healthy eating.

Although my sought-after "return to normal" has not materialized, I am deeply grateful. I have learned so much, gained so much knowledge and maybe a little wisdom. I learned a new definition of hope—*our only opportunity for control*. That real, open-hearted connection is critical; that gratitude is one of our greatest tools; and that being of service is one of our greatest gifts. I learned to never stop trying and to never give up. I learned to appreciate every day, and work to be present and conscious in the moment.

I have so much—my family who inspires me every day, my dedicated teachers who continue to support me, the people who allow me to be of service in their lives, my daily practices, and the many, many aspects of love. All these help me to continuously create and shape a life I love and am passionate about even when I am in pain. I learned we never really know what the next moment or twenty-four years have in store for us; however, with our minds and our practices, we can make it something special.

How to Use This Book

You can start this journal at the beginning or open to any page. This is your journal—you should do it your way. While this is not a long book, it might take some time to get through it. Approach it as a practice. Commit to a page a day, or pick a day of the week and complete a few pages. Allow yourself to be in the moment as you interact with each page, each prompt, each activity. Engage with this journal when you feel lighthearted and when you feel downhearted. The tools you'll learn can make the bright times brighter and the dark times lighter.

I know because I use them every day.

*You can do small things inside
your mind that will lead to
big changes in your brain
and your experience of living.*
—Rick Hanson

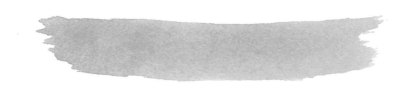

The secret of health for both mind and body is not to mourn for the past, worry about the future, or anticipate troubles, but to live in the present moment wisely and earnestly.

—Buddha

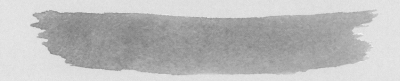

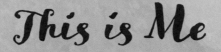

This is Me

Recognizing, acknowledging, and recording what we like about ourselves and our lives helps train our brains to focus on what is working for us, what we are enjoying, and things that contribute to experiencing happiness. On these next pages, capture your thoughts about yourself and your life.

QUALITIES THAT DESCRIBE ME...

Circle the words that describe the qualities you see in yourself and the qualities you'd like to see in yourself. How you are now, and how you'd like to be. Use the empty space to include additional qualities that are important to you.

Thoughtful

HIGH INTEGRITY   Resilient

Blessed   Healthy   KIND

PEACEFUL   Sensitive

INSIGHTFUL   Funny   Loving

Endearing   COMMITTED

Problem Solver   Optimist

Humorous   WISE   GIVING

Engaging   Imaginative

COMPASSIONATE   STRONG

PROSPEROUS   One-of-a-Kind

Courageous   INSPIRING   Grateful

Gentle   JOYFUL

THOUGHTS THAT DESCRIBE ME...

New discoveries in neuroscience are uncovering the importance of thoughts, how they trigger physical, emotional, and mental responses in our bodies, impacting overall health. Fill out the sentences using the words you selected on the previous page to describe yourself and how you see yourself growing. Read and reread these sentences every day to help create and support your positive well-being.

I AM STRONG, RESILIENT, AND GRATEFUL.

I AM _____

I AM _____

I AM _____

I AM _____

I AM _____

Describe what you'd like your life to be filled with using the words on the previous page.

MY LIFE IS FULL OF ABUNDANCE AND PROSPERITY.

MY LIFE IS _____

MY WORK IS _____

MY FAMILY IS _____

MY FRIENDS ARE _____

MY COMMUNITY IS _____

MY HOME IS _____

MY LOVES

Take some time and think about all the people, places, and things you love. List them below to revisit whenever you want or when you need a pick-me-up.

I LOVE _____

I LOVE _____

I LOVE _____

I LOVE _____

I LOVE _____

I LOVE _____

I LOVE _____

I LOVE _____

I LOVE _____

I LOVE _____

MY FAVORITES

Capture anything and everything that falls into the category of favorites and that you have fond memories around. It could be family, friends, stories, foods, books, writers, poets, musicians, songs, bands, movies, shows, theatre, restaurants, vacations, and more, just as long as it holds the title of "My Favorite."

MY FAVORITE _____ IS _____

MY FAVORITE _____ IS _____

MY FAVORITE _____ IS _____

MY FAVORITE _____ IS _____

MY FAVORITE _____ IS _____

MY FAVORITE _____ IS _____

MY FAVORITE _____ IS _____

MY FAVORITE _____ IS _____

MY FAVORITE _____ IS _____

MY FAVORITE _____ IS _____

MY SPECIAL MEMORIES

Capture your stories about special moments, events, and experiences that always make you smile.

I REMEMBER FEELING SO HAPPY WHEN:

_____

_____

_____

_____

_____

I REMEMBER FEELING SO CARED FOR WHEN:

_____

_____

_____

_____

_____

I REMEMBER FEELING SO LOVED WHEN:

_____

_____

_____

_____

_____

I REMEMBER FEELING SO JOYFUL WHEN:

_____

_____

_____

_____

_____

THINGS I LIKE ABOUT MYSELF

This is your private space, so don't be shy capturing all your amazing traits and things you do well.

I LIKE MY _____

I LIKE MY _____

I LIKE MY _____

I LIKE MY _____

I LIKE MY _____

I LIKE MY _____

I LIKE MY _____

I LIKE MY _____

I LIKE MY _____

I LIKE MY _____

1) I AM GOOD AT _____
_____

2) I AM GOOD AT _____
_____

3) I AM GOOD AT _____
_____

4) I AM GOOD AT _____
_____

5) I AM GOOD AT _____
_____

6) I AM GOOD AT _____
_____

7) I AM GOOD AT _____
_____

8) I AM GOOD AT _____
_____

9) I AM GOOD AT _____
_____

10) I AM GOOD AT _____
_____

I BELIEVE I CAN...

When dealing with chronic pain and illness, it is important to identify activities you want to do and envision yourself doing them. List those actions below.

I BELIEVE I CAN _____

I BELIEVE I CAN _____

I BELIEVE I CAN _____

I BELIEVE I CAN _____

I BELIEVE I CAN _____

I BELIEVE I CAN _____

I BELIEVE I CAN _____

I BELIEVE I CAN _____

I BELIEVE I CAN _____

I BELIEVE I CAN _____

I BELIEVE I CAN _____

I AM COMMITTED TO...

List those endeavors you are going to diligently pursue.

- _____
  _____
  _____

- _____
  _____
  _____

- _____
  _____
  _____

- _____
  _____
  _____

- _____
  _____

Gratitude unlocks the fullness of life. It turns what we have into enough, and more. It turns denial into acceptance, chaos to order, confusion to clarity. It can turn a meal into a feast, a house into a home, a stranger into a friend... Gratitude makes sense of our past, brings peace for today, and creates a vision for tomorrow.

—Melody Beattie

The Power of Gratitude

The power of gratitude is almost incomprehensible as it seems to be such a simple act of acknowledgment. Gratitude has the ability to help us melt away challenges by positively shifting our perspective, enhancing our well-being, and building resiliency. It is critical to understand that gratitude is not just a feeling; it is a tool that brings peace, even happiness, when confronting pain and loss. In fact, studies show gratitude can be used to help with mood swings, anxiety, and post-traumatic stress.

Since gratitude is a state of being and not an emotion, generating and repeating gratitude statements is helpful when you're upset, angry, or hurt as well as when you are happy. You can express gratitude over things that have happened. You can also express gratitude over things you would like to happen. These are called gratitude intentions. There is not a right way or wrong way to be grateful or to do gratitude.

However, gratitude is not always easy. When facing overwhelming difficulties, pain, and deep loss, reaching for gratitude can feel more challenging than climbing Mount Everest. According to Dr. Robert Emmons at the University of California, Davis, gratitude is a choice: "It means that we sharpen our ability to recognize and acknowledge the giftedness of life. It means that we make a conscious decision to see blessings instead of curses. It means that our internal reactions are not determined by external forces. That gratitude is a conscious decision does not imply that it is an easy decision... while gratitude is pleasant, it is not easy."

IN MY EVERYDAY LIFE I AM GRATEFUL FOR...

Creating a gratitude practice by journaling daily gratitudes or writing daily gratitude lists helps build resiliency; and on those really hard days you can read and reread your gratitudes from previous days. Gratitude is most powerful when it becomes part of your daily routine.

I AM GRATEFUL FOR _____

I AM GRATEFUL FOR _____

I AM GRATEFUL FOR _____

I AM GRATEFUL FOR _____

I AM GRATEFUL FOR _____

I AM GRATEFUL FOR _____

I AM GRATEFUL FOR _____

I AM GRATEFUL FOR _____

I AM GRATEFUL FOR _____

I AM GRATEFUL FOR _____

SPECIAL EVERYDAY MOMENTS
I AM GRATEFUL FOR...

I AM GRATEFUL FOR _____

I AM GRATEFUL FOR _____

I AM GRATEFUL FOR _____

I AM GRATEFUL FOR _____

I AM GRATEFUL FOR _____

I AM GRATEFUL FOR _____

I AM GRATEFUL FOR _____

I AM GRATEFUL FOR _____

I AM GRATEFUL FOR _____

I AM GRATEFUL FOR _____

IN MY HOME I AM GRATEFUL FOR...

I AM GRATEFUL FOR _____

I AM GRATEFUL FOR _____

I AM GRATEFUL FOR _____

I AM GRATEFUL FOR _____

I AM GRATEFUL FOR _____

I AM GRATEFUL FOR _____

I AM GRATEFUL FOR _____

I AM GRATEFUL FOR _____

I AM GRATEFUL FOR _____

I AM GRATEFUL FOR _____

ACTIVITIES I LIKE TO DO
THAT I AM GRATEFUL FOR...

I AM GRATEFUL FOR _____

I AM GRATEFUL FOR _____

I AM GRATEFUL FOR _____

I AM GRATEFUL FOR _____

I AM GRATEFUL FOR _____

I AM GRATEFUL FOR _____

I AM GRATEFUL FOR _____

I AM GRATEFUL FOR _____

I AM GRATEFUL FOR _____

I AM GRATEFUL FOR _____

FAMILY & FRIENDS I AM GRATEFUL FOR...

I AM GRATEFUL FOR _____

I AM GRATEFUL FOR _____

I AM GRATEFUL FOR _____

I AM GRATEFUL FOR _____

I AM GRATEFUL FOR _____

I AM GRATEFUL FOR _____

I AM GRATEFUL FOR _____

I AM GRATEFUL FOR _____

I AM GRATEFUL FOR _____

I AM GRATEFUL FOR _____

FAMILY & FRIENDS I AM GRATEFUL FOR...

I AM GRATEFUL FOR _____

I AM GRATEFUL FOR _____

I AM GRATEFUL FOR _____

I AM GRATEFUL FOR _____

I AM GRATEFUL FOR _____

I AM GRATEFUL FOR _____

I AM GRATEFUL FOR _____

I AM GRATEFUL FOR _____

I AM GRATEFUL FOR _____

I AM GRATEFUL FOR _____

NEIGHBORS, COLLEAGUES, HEALTH CARE PRACTITIONERS, COMMUNITY MEMBERS, AND OTHER PEOPLE IN MY LIFE I AM GRATEFUL FOR...

I AM GRATEFUL FOR _____

I AM GRATEFUL FOR _____

I AM GRATEFUL FOR _____

I AM GRATEFUL FOR _____

I AM GRATEFUL FOR _____

I AM GRATEFUL FOR _____

I AM GRATEFUL FOR _____

I AM GRATEFUL FOR _____

I AM GRATEFUL FOR _____

I AM GRATEFUL FOR _____

NEIGHBORS, COLLEAGUES, HEALTH CARE PRACTITIONERS, COMMUNITY MEMBERS, AND OTHER PEOPLE IN MY LIFE I AM GRATEFUL FOR...

I AM GRATEFUL FOR _____

I AM GRATEFUL FOR _____

I AM GRATEFUL FOR _____

I AM GRATEFUL FOR _____

I AM GRATEFUL FOR _____

I AM GRATEFUL FOR _____

I AM GRATEFUL FOR _____

I AM GRATEFUL FOR _____

I AM GRATEFUL FOR _____

I AM GRATEFUL FOR _____

THANK YOU TO...

Consider the many gifts, acts of kindness, and support you have received in your life. Say thank you to these people now. Write down the names of the people who generously gave to you, and what their contributions meant to you.

THANK YOU TO _____ FOR

_____

_____

THANK YOU TO _____ FOR

_____

_____

THANK YOU TO _____ FOR

_____

_____

THANK YOU TO _____ FOR

_____

_____

THANK YOU TO _____ FOR

_____

_____

THANK YOU TO _____ FOR

_____

_____

THANK YOU TO _____ FOR

_____

_____

THANK YOU TO _____ FOR

_____

_____

THANK YOU TO _____ FOR

_____

_____

GRATITUDE INTENTIONS

These gratitude lists are different from the ones you just completed. Here, you will complete gratitude statements for what you desire in your life as if it currently exists. For example, if you are looking for a new place to live, you would write: *I am grateful for my new home.* Reread your gratitude intentions regularly and keep adding to them over time.

I AM GRATEFUL FOR _____

I AM GRATEFUL FOR _____

I AM GRATEFUL FOR _____

I AM GRATEFUL FOR _____

I AM GRATEFUL FOR _____

I AM GRATEFUL FOR _____

I AM GRATEFUL FOR _____

I AM GRATEFUL FOR _____

I AM GRATEFUL FOR _____

I AM GRATEFUL FOR _____

I AM GRATEFUL FOR _____

I AM GRATEFUL FOR _____

I AM GRATEFUL FOR _____

I AM GRATEFUL FOR _____

I AM GRATEFUL FOR _____

I AM GRATEFUL FOR _____

I AM GRATEFUL FOR _____

I AM GRATEFUL FOR _____

I AM GRATEFUL FOR _____

I AM GRATEFUL FOR _____

I AM GRATEFUL FOR _____

I AM GRATEFUL FOR _____

I AM GRATEFUL FOR _____

I AM GRATEFUL FOR _____

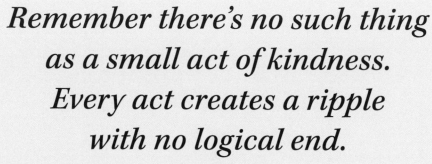

Remember there's no such thing as a small act of kindness. Every act creates a ripple with no logical end.

—Scott Adams

The Joys of Kindness & Connection

Kindness and connection are gifts that can be easily given and received every day. It can be as simple as a smile at a stranger, a check-in on a neighbor, or a quick text to a friend. Each of these efforts takes only a few minutes, but they have the power to change someone's day, including your own. Whether you are extending or accepting a helping hand, the warmth, the happiness, and even joy are always present. So, share yourself, your kindness—you will feel better.

Fill these pages out in one day or over many days, whatever you are able to do. Recount the kindnesses you shared and received recently.

TODAY I WAS KIND TO:

-
-
-
-
-
-
-
-
-

TODAY THESE PEOPLE WERE KIND TO ME:

-
-
-
-
-
-
-
-
-

RECENTLY, I GAVE...

Fill in the lines with your acts of generosity. How was the act received, and how did that make you feel?

I GAVE _____ TO _____

IT FELT GOOD AS THEY RESPONDED BY _____

_____

I GAVE _____ TO _____

IT FELT GOOD AS THEY RESPONDED BY _____

_____

I GAVE _____ TO _____

IT FELT GOOD AS THEY RESPONDED BY _____

_____

I GAVE _____ TO _____

IT FELT GOOD AS THEY RESPONDED BY _____

_____

I GAVE _____ TO _____

IT FELT GOOD AS THEY RESPONDED BY _____

_____

RECENTLY, I RECEIVED...

Fill in the lines describing your receiving acts of generosity. Who shared their generosity, and how did you feel?

_____ GAVE ME _____

IT FELT GOOD AND I RESPONDED BY _____

_____

_____ GAVE ME _____

IT FELT GOOD AND I RESPONDED BY _____

_____

_____ GAVE ME _____

IT FELT GOOD AND I RESPONDED BY _____

_____

_____ GAVE ME _____

IT FELT GOOD AND I RESPONDED BY _____

_____

_____ GAVE ME _____

IT FELT GOOD AND I RESPONDED BY _____

_____

On these pages, recall being the recipient of acts of warmheartedness. Capture your memories and how you felt. Revisit these pages when you need a mental, emotional, or physical pick-me-up.

KINDNESSES I REMEMBER:

-
-
-
-
-
-
-
-
-

KINDNESSES THAT TOUCHED MY HEART:

-
-
-
-
-
-
-
-
-

Despite all the technological ways to instantly transfer information to one another, people are self-reporting increased feelings of loneliness, isolation, and difficulties with communication. One of the most generous gifts we can give to anyone is to authentically and completely listen to them. Below, list the conversations you remember where you listened attentively.

I LISTENED CLOSELY TO _____

WHEN THEY TALKED ABOUT _____

I LISTENED CLOSELY TO _____

WHEN THEY TALKED ABOUT _____

I LISTENED CLOSELY TO _____

WHEN THEY TALKED ABOUT _____

I LISTENED CLOSELY TO _____

WHEN THEY TALKED ABOUT _____

I LISTENED CLOSELY TO _____

WHEN THEY TALKED ABOUT _____

I LISTENED CLOSELY TO _____

WHEN THEY TALKED ABOUT _____

I LISTENED CLOSELY TO _____

WHEN THEY TALKED ABOUT _____

The feeling of someone really listening and taking in what we are saying is a loving gift. Recall conversations in which you felt authentically heard and how it made you feel.

_____ REALLY HEARD ME WHEN
I WAS TALKING ABOUT _____
BEING LISTENED TO CLOSELY, I FELT _____

_____ REALLY HEARD ME WHEN
I WAS TALKING ABOUT _____
BEING LISTENED TO CLOSELY, I FELT _____

_____ REALLY HEARD ME WHEN
I WAS TALKING ABOUT _____
BEING LISTENED TO CLOSELY, I FELT _____

_____ REALLY HEARD ME WHEN
I WAS TALKING ABOUT _____
BEING LISTENED TO CLOSELY, I FELT _____

_____ REALLY HEARD ME WHEN
I WAS TALKING ABOUT _____
BEING LISTENED TO CLOSELY, I FELT _____

_____ REALLY HEARD ME WHEN
I WAS TALKING ABOUT _____
BEING LISTENED TO CLOSELY, I FELT _____

Research reveals that staying connected to others plays a significant role in maintaining health and well-being. List people you connect with regularly. For example: *I connect with Faith every day.* Also, list those you'd like to communicate with more frequently and how you plan to reach out to them. The people you would like to reconnect with and how. For example: *I'd like to connect with Thomas more. I will reach out by text.*

I CONNECT WITH _____

HOW OFTER (OR WHEN) _____

I CONNECT WITH _____

HOW OFTER (OR WHEN) _____

I'D LIKE TO CONNECT WITH _____

I WILL REACH OUT BY _____

I'D LIKE TO CONNECT WITH _____

I WILL REACH OUT BY _____

I'D LIKE TO RECONNECT WITH _____

I WILL REACH OUT BY _____

I'D LIKE TO RECONNECT WITH _____

I WILL REACH OUT BY _____

Think of the people and places that provide us with familiarity and comfort. Write down these comforts below.

PLACES WHERE I REGULARLY GO AND I'M KNOWN:

_____

_____

_____

_____

_____

OTHER PEOPLE AND PLACES WHO ARE PART OF MY COMMUNITY:

_____

_____

_____

_____

_____

*When we give to others
from the heart, we receive
as much in return.*
—Kahlil Gibran

The Benefits of Service

Assisting others and engaging in something that is bigger than ourselves can provide purpose in our lives. When we give to others from the heart, we receive as much as in return. Unexpected joy breaks through even during the most challenging times to keep us going. Research suggests that being of service also helps the mind and body heal as well as assists with recovery.

Capture your acts of service to loved ones, the community, and strangers.

TODAY, I WAS ABLE TO HELP _____
BY _____

TODAY, I WAS ABLE TO HELP _____
BY _____

TODAY, I WAS ABLE TO HELP _____
BY _____

TODAY, I WAS ABLE TO HELP _____
BY _____

RECENTLY, I WAS ABLE TO HELP _____
BY _____

RECENTLY, I WAS ABLE TO HELP _____
BY _____

RECENTLY, I WAS ABLE TO HELP _____
BY _____

RECENTLY, I WAS ABLE TO HELP _____
BY _____

Having a purpose and being of service to others can positively affect how we feel emotionally, mentally, and even physically. Think about situations when you were helping someone else. Write about how you felt before, during, and after you were of service.

_____

_____

_____

_____

_____

_____

_____

_____

_____

_____

_____

_____

_____

_____

_____

_____

_____

_____

Write about all those caring, beautiful things you do for others that make a difference in their lives. For example: *Every Monday I bring a fresh muffin to my neighbor and we talk for a while.*

I MAKE A DIFFERENCE BY _____

_____

_____

I MAKE A DIFFERENCE BY _____

_____

_____

I MAKE A DIFFERENCE BY _____

_____

_____

I MAKE A DIFFERENCE BY _____

_____

_____

I MAKE A DIFFERENCE BY _____

_____

_____

On this page, write down many of the things you do to selflessly help each other. For example: *I spend 3 hours a week collecting food for the food pantry.*

I AM OF SERVICE TO _____

I AM OF SERVICE TO _____

I AM OF SERVICE TO _____

I AM OF SERVICE TO _____

I AM OF SERVICE TO _____

I AM OF SERVICE TO _____

I AM OF SERVICE TO _____

I AM OF SERVICE TO _____

I AM OF SERVICE TO _____

I AM OF SERVICE TO _____

Daily we make contributions to others, and most often we don't even realize it. Use this space to recognize yourself for many of the things you do to be of service. You can include anything from a monetary donation to an impactful cause, to listening to a friend going through a difficult time.

I CONTRIBUTE TO _____

I CONTRIBUTE TO _____

I CONTRIBUTE TO _____

I CONTRIBUTE TO _____

I CONTRIBUTE TO _____

I CONTRIBUTE TO _____

I CONTRIBUTE TO _____

I CONTRIBUTE TO _____

I CONTRIBUTE TO _____

I CONTRIBUTE TO _____

THESE ARE THE THINGS I DO TO BRING OTHERS JOY:

-
-
-
-
-
-
-
-
-
-

Sometimes contributions are made through participation in community groups and organizations.

THESE ARE GROUPS I AM AND HAVE BEEN INVOLVED WITH:

-
-
-
-
-

THESE ARE ORGANIZATIONS I BELONG TO:

-
-
-
-
-

You must do the thing you think you cannot do.

—Eleanor Roosevelt

The Importance of Movement

For those of us in pain, exercise and movement can be especially difficult. The paradox is our bodies need to move, but the pain says stop. Our own bodies are giving us mixed messages. So, the question becomes: what should we do? This is a uniquely challenging question as all of us are different. We have our own restrictions, our own pain, and our own paths. Therefore, we have to tailor our physical activities to our own needs and customize our exercise programs. However, what most of us can do is spend five minutes a day moving a part of our bodies, creating a daily practice of movement. Research supports this action in that it will help create new neuropathways and build resilience—something we all can use.

DAILY PRACTICES

List physical activities you do every day, from moving around your home to taking a walk outside. Now, congratulate yourself! Over the next week, add one or more new movements to your list.

- _____
- _____
- _____
- _____
- _____
- _____
- _____
- _____
- _____
- _____
- _____
- _____
- _____

ONE DAY AT A TIME

Moving isn't easy for everyone. Create a movement list for the next two weeks by committing to at least one physical activity per day for the next fourteen days.

DAY	ACTIVITY	DAY	ACTIVITY
1		8	
2		9	
3		10	
4		11	
5		12	
6		13	
7		14	

BREATH

Breathing is such a natural thing. For the most part, it just happens without us having to think about it. For two weeks, spend some time every day quietly watching your breath.

Sit or lie in a comfortable position. Set a timer for five minutes. Close your eyes. Observe your breath. Are you breathing through your nose or mouth? Are your inhalations deep or shallow? Are the exhalations the same quality as the inhalations? Keep focused, watching your breathing until the timer goes off.

Capture what you noticed.

DAY	OBSERVATIONS	DAY	OBSERVATIONS
1		8	
2		9	
3		10	
4		11	
5		12	
6		13	
7		14	

MEDITATION

Developing a meditation practice can be life affirming, and there are many approaches to meditation. Here is a short, accessible meditation for you to engage.

First, find a comfortable place to lie down or to sit upright for five minutes.

Get comfortably situated and set a timer for five minutes.

Close your eyes. Notice your breath. Observe your breathing for five inhalations and five exhalations.

Now picture in your mind's eye a beautiful, serene, and quiet place. A place you feel safe and protected. Settle into that space and breath.

When your timer goes off, gently open your eyes. Take a few minutes to reorient to your current space. Slowly rise.

DAILY ROUTINES CHART

Fill in what a normal week looks like for you. Record your regular activities.

	SUNDAY	MONDAY	TUESDAY
Morning			
Afternoon			
Evening			

WEDNESDAY	THURSDAY	FRIDAY	SATURDAY

IDEAL DAILY ROUTINES CHART

Create what you'd like to have your normal week look like. Consider what activities you would add to or remove from the previous chart, and make those changes.

	SUNDAY	MONDAY	TUESDAY
Morning			
Afternoon			
Evening			

WEDNESDAY	THURSDAY	FRIDAY	SATURDAY

WHEN I CAN DO MORE, I LIKE TO...

List what you enjoy doing when you're having
a good day.

- _____
- _____
- _____
- _____
- _____
- _____
- _____
- _____
- _____
- _____
- _____
- _____
- _____

WHEN I NEED A BREAK, I LIKE TO...

List what you do to self-care on challenging days.

- _____
- _____
- _____
- _____
- _____
- _____
- _____
- _____
- _____
- _____
- _____
- _____
- _____

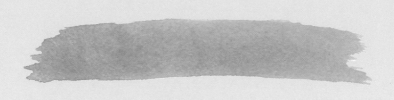

*...everything in life responds
to the song of the heart.*
—Ernest Holmes

The Consciousness of Creativity

The act of being creative is another one of those powerful gifts that is often misunderstood. We grow up believing we need to have "talent" to create. However, being creative is not about the end result; it is about the act itself. Releasing ourselves into creativity allows us to regenerate, relax, regroup, and even relieve pain, making it a favorite resiliency tool.

BEING CREATIVE

Circle creative activities that you like to do individually and with others. If there is something you enjoy that isn't on the list, add it!

- Coloring inside the lines
- Coloring outside the lines
- Acting
- Painting
- Collaging
- Dancing
- Singing
- Sewing
- Printmaking
- Baking

- Cake decorating
- Storytelling
- Drawing
- Writing
- Sketching
- Filmmaking
- Photography
- Gardening
- Reading
- Scrapbooking

Identify one to three activities from the previous page that you would like to do regularly, even daily. List those activities below and write why you are drawn to each activity.

1)

2)

3)

Now, choose a project you would like to do or something you've always wanted to try. You can make it as simple or elaborate as you want. Remember, it is the act of creating that is most valuable; the end product is the bonus. Generate your own project or select a project from the list.

- Make a family photobook
- Make a collage
- Create a painting
- Paint furniture
- Write a story
- Bake cookies, pastries, or pies
- Write poetry
- Plant a garden
- Conduct a science experiment
- Compose an original song
- Write your family story
- Create a cookbook

Start the creative process by jotting down your thoughts and ideas about your project. Outline the materials you need and how you are going to procure them. Pick a date to get started as soon as you can, and enjoy creating.

_____

_____

_____

_____

_____

_____

_____

_____

_____

_____

_____

_____

_____

START DATE _____

BEING CREATIVE EVERYDAY

It doesn't matter if you are working on your creative project or doing something totally unrelated, just do something creative every day for at least five minutes. You can sing a song, do a dance, color, write a letter, cook a meal, or more. Fill in this daily chart with creative activities from your list and check off each day that you do something creative.

CREATIVE ACTIVITY	DATE	DONE ✓

CREATIVE ACTIVITY	DATE	DONE ✓

COLOR WITH ABANDON

Grab a pencil, a crayon, a marker, or a pen and color these two pages any way you desire.

You can scribble, draw, or sketch. Relax, breathe, and go! Have fun expressing yourself in this moment.

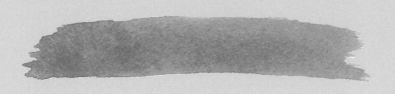

*Your vision will become
clear only when you look
into your heart.
Who looks outside, dreams.
Who looks inside, awakens.*

—Carl Jung

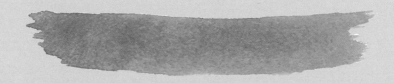

The Peace of Quiet Moments

In this world that is moving faster than ever with constant distractions vying for our attention, many of us have forgotten how to embrace the quiet. To sit serenely and watch a sunset. To meditate or pray before we rise. Savor our food as we eat a meal. Listen to our favorite music or really engage with a piece of artwork. Most of us need to relearn this skill as we are out of practice. Spend five minutes each day being still and observe what happens.

It is in appreciating the everyday that we can find peace, solace, contentment, and even relief from our challenges.

FROM TODAY I WANT TO REMEMBER
_____

FROM TODAY I WANT TO REMEMBER
_____

FROM TODAY I WANT TO REMEMBER
_____

FROM TODAY I WANT TO REMEMBER
_____

FROM TODAY I WANT TO REMEMBER
_____

FROM TODAY I WANT TO REMEMBER
_____

FROM TODAY I WANT TO REMEMBER
_____

FROM TODAY I WANT TO REMEMBER
_____

FROM TODAY I WANT TO REMEMBER
_____

FROM TODAY I WANT TO REMEMBER
_____

FROM TODAY I WANT TO REMEMBER

_____

FROM TODAY I WANT TO REMEMBER

_____

FROM TODAY I WANT TO REMEMBER

_____

FROM TODAY I WANT TO REMEMBER

_____

FROM TODAY I WANT TO REMEMBER

_____

FROM TODAY I WANT TO REMEMBER

_____

FROM TODAY I WANT TO REMEMBER

_____

FROM TODAY I WANT TO REMEMBER

_____

FROM TODAY I WANT TO REMEMBER

_____

Make it a regular practice to pause and observe the world around you. Take note of things that make you think, smile, and laugh.

TODAY I NOTICED:

_____

_____

_____

_____

_____

_____

_____

_____

TODAY I WATCHED:

_____

_____

_____

_____

_____

_____

_____

_____

_____

MUSINGS & OBSERVATIONS

These pages are for you to capture complete and
incomplete ideas, thoughts, and insights to keep and
build on.

_____

_____

_____

_____

_____

_____

_____

_____

_____

_____

_____

_____

_____

_____

_____

MUSINGS & OBSERVATIONS

When you hold resentment toward another, you are bound to that person or condition by an emotional link that is stronger than steel. Forgiveness is the only way to dissolve that link and get free.

—Catherine Ponder

The Art of Forgiveness

Forgiveness is another one of those incredibly simple and powerful tools. It is a gift to each and every one of us. First, we must learn to forgive ourselves. If we don't learn to forgive ourselves, it is difficult for us to learn to forgive others. The most interesting part of forgiveness is that it is often thought of as something you do for someone else. Well, that is only part of it—because forgiveness is also a gift to oneself. Forgiving someone does not excuse the transgression; however, it frees us from continuing to carry the hurt, anger, and upset with us, allowing us to heal and move on. As we master the art of forgiveness, we will find ourselves less encumbered by the small and large upsets of life.

Fill these two pages with experiences to release and let go of.

I RELEASE _____

I RELEASE _____

I RELEASE _____

I RELEASE _____

I RELEASE _____

I RELEASE _____

I RELEASE _____

I RELEASE _____

I RELEASE _____

I RELEASE _____

I RELEASE _____

I RELEASE _____

I RELEASE _____

I RELEASE _____

I RELEASE _____

I RELEASE _____

I RELEASE _____

I RELEASE _____

I RELEASE _____

I RELEASE _____

We all have things we wish we could undo, change, or take back. Have compassion for yourself, release your regrets, and forgive yourself. Use these pages as a safe place for you to let go.

I FORGIVE MYSELF FOR _____

I FORGIVE MYSELF FOR _____

I FORGIVE MYSELF FOR _____

I FORGIVE MYSELF FOR _____

I FORGIVE MYSELF FOR _____

I FORGIVE MYSELF FOR _____

I FORGIVE MYSELF FOR _____

I FORGIVE MYSELF FOR _____

I FORGIVE MYSELF FOR _____

I FORGIVE MYSELF FOR _____

I FORGIVE MYSELF FOR _____

I FORGIVE MYSELF FOR _____

I FORGIVE MYSELF FOR _____

I FORGIVE MYSELF FOR _____

I FORGIVE MYSELF FOR _____

I FORGIVE MYSELF FOR _____

I FORGIVE MYSELF FOR _____

I FORGIVE MYSELF FOR _____

I FORGIVE MYSELF FOR _____

I FORGIVE MYSELF FOR _____

Fill out these next pages in one sitting or over time. Remember that when you forgive, you are releasing the anger, hurt, and harm that you received. You are saying you will no longer carry the pain with me. "I forgive you" means "I release myself from the pain you caused me." You can keep your forgiveness thoughts and statements private, or you can share them with those you forgive. It is completely your choice.

I FORGIVE _____

I FORGIVE _____

I FORGIVE _____

I FORGIVE _____

I FORGIVE _____

I FORGIVE _____

I FORGIVE _____

I FORGIVE _____

I FORGIVE _____

I FORGIVE _____

I FORGIVE _____

I FORGIVE _____

I FORGIVE _____

I FORGIVE _____

I FORGIVE _____

I FORGIVE _____

I FORGIVE _____

I FORGIVE _____

I FORGIVE _____

I FORGIVE _____

These final forgiveness pages are for you to note any people you'd like to forgive you.

This exercise is just for you, so open your heart and allow it to heal.

_____ FORGIVES ME

_____ FORGIVES ME

_____ FORGIVES ME

_____ FORGIVES ME

_____ FORGIVES ME

_____ FORGIVES ME

_____ FORGIVES ME

_____ FORGIVES ME

_____ FORGIVES ME

_____ FORGIVES ME

_____ FORGIVES ME

_____ FORGIVES ME

_____ FORGIVES ME

_____ FORGIVES ME

_____ FORGIVES ME

_____ FORGIVES ME

_____ FORGIVES ME

_____ FORGIVES ME

_____ FORGIVES ME

_____ FORGIVES ME

We must accept finite disappointment, but never lose infinite hope.

—Martin Luther King

For the Hard Days

All of us who have experienced chronic pain or illness know these days all too well. When the pain, the challenges from the condition, the feelings of aloneness, or a combination of those three just gets heavy. All the resiliency tools and practices in this journal are designed to assist on these difficult days. However, some days generating anything can be too hard. So, this section does much of the generation for you.

Travel through these pages in any order that calls you. Start at the beginning of the section, or open to any page and go from there. Sometimes it will take just a few pages to feel a positive shift. Other times you may find you go through the section multiple times. There is not a right or wrong way to do this work; the helpful part is to engage with the practices.

GRATITUDE STATEMENTS

Read these gratitude statements out loud or in your head. Sometimes you might read a few quickly, and other times you may repeat all of them multiple times. Often people report how difficult it is to get started. They are sure they can only do one statement, then find themselves doing thirty or more. Honor yourself and wherever you are today! Use the free space to add any of your favorite gratitude statements to the list.

- I am grateful for joy.
- I am grateful for my determination.
- I am grateful for my sense of humor.
- I am grateful for my friends.
- I am grateful for my family.
- I am grateful for seeing the good in others.
- I am grateful for good jokes.
- I am grateful for all acts of kindness.
- I am grateful to be able to help others.
- I am grateful for keeping my cool today.
- I am grateful for the vitality I have.
- I am grateful for a hearty laugh.
- I am grateful for my favorite foods.
- I am grateful for books to read and movies to watch.

- I am grateful for every day.
- I am grateful for all the beauty in the world.
- I am grateful for the sunrise.
- I am grateful for a gorgeous sky.
- I am grateful for fresh air.
- I am grateful for a warm breeze.
- I am grateful for a sunny day.
- I am grateful for time outdoors.
- I am grateful for the oceans.
- I am grateful for the mountains.
- I am grateful for the forests.
- I am grateful for the sunset.
- I am grateful for peaceful moments.
- I am grateful for genuine caring.

- _____
- _____
- _____
- _____
- _____
- _____

GRATITUDE STATEMENTS

Add any of your special gratitude statements to the list.

- I am grateful for today.
- I am grateful for my life.
- I am grateful for my healing.
- I am grateful for my resilience.
- I am grateful for my talents.
- I am grateful for being able to be me.
- I am grateful for feeling better now.
- I am grateful for having faith in myself.
- I am grateful for having the strength to never give up.
- I am grateful for my courage to reach for the stars.
- I am grateful for my hopes and dreams.
- I am grateful for those who support me.
- I am grateful for the smiles I receive.

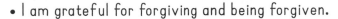

- I am grateful for forgiving and being forgiven.
- I am grateful for pursuing my dreams.
- I am grateful for learning new lessons.
- I am grateful for seeing the positive.
- I am grateful for being of service.
- I am grateful for abundance.
- I am grateful for new experiences.
- I am grateful for a gentle hug.
- I am grateful for others understanding without needing explanation.
- I am grateful for today's opportunities.
- I am grateful for dreams of fancy.
- I am grateful for creativity and imagination.
- I am grateful for peaceful moments.

- _____
- _____
- _____
- _____
- _____
- _____

PERSONAL STATEMENTS

These statements work just like the gratitude statements, but are even more personal. They reflect positive feelings we have or would like to have about ourselves. Research reveals our thoughts affect our well-being, so read the statements below. Repeating them over and over can help build new plasticity and resilience.

- I am loved.
- I love myself as I am now.
- I accept myself.
- I forgive myself.
- I release my fears.
- I laugh every day.
- I am free to enjoy.
- I am heard and respected.
- I am open to new experiences.
- I give to and receive from my community.
- I am peaceful.

- My past is complete.
- My thoughts shape my experiences.
- I notice the many rainbows on my path.
- I listen with an open heart.
- I find the calm in the storm.
- I build strength every day.
- I imagine inspiring possibilities.
- I easily share with others.
- I discover peace in the moment.
- My day ends in gratitude.
- We are all connected.

THINGS I CAN DO TO HELP MYSELF FEEL BETTER

When our "new normal" includes dealing with daily pain and health issues, it can be challenging to keep ourselves moving during the hard days. You know, those days that really take it out of you. The activities on these pages can assist you during those difficult times, even during those dark moments. Begin with the one that calls to you most. If nothing is really speaking to you, start at the top of the list.

1) *Create something—anything.* Sing a song, make a favorite snack or meal, paint, color, write, send a humorous text to a friend or play an instrument. It is the act of creating, making something that didn't exist the moment before, that can help you feel better. Stay in the act of creating and notice the peace and lack of judgment.

2) *Play or be silly, or both.* Allow that childlike enthusiasm to surface and guide you into doing something just to do it. Something that you enjoy and makes you laugh. It does not have to be clever or sophisticated, it just has to be fun for you in the moment.

3) *Smile at least five times today.* If there are other people around, smile at them. Observe the power of the smile, both for you and for the recipient of the smile.

4) *Treat yourself.* Give yourself a gift, something you love that brings joy to you. It can be a favorite cup of tea or something more elaborate, as long as it is easy for you to do right now. It is the act of treating yourself that has a bigger, more positive impact on you than the actual gift.

5) *Spend time with someone you care about.* This can be in person, over the phone, or virtually. Set up time to connect today.

6) *Eat healthily.* It may sound simple, but it works. Give your body the nutrients it needs, and it will respond gratefully.

7) *Exercise.* (You knew this one was coming!) Even on the hard days, it is really important to move. If it is for just five minutes, that's great—as long as the body is active in some way. If you set aside a certain time every day for movement, it will make it easier.

8) *Be open to new things.* Investigate something you have always wanted to do but haven't done.

9) *Forgive* someone or an organization you felt treated you wrongly.

10) *Help someone else today.* It is remarkable how being of service helps us feel better in the moment.

SMILE... CHUCKLE... LAUGH... LAUGH HARD

It is amazing how healing a smile, a chuckle, and laughing hard can be in the moment and over time. When we learn to laugh as a favorite tool, it opens doors to joy when they were previously closed by pain or fear. So sometimes we just have to focus on smiling and laughing. Let's get started.

I found myself smiling when:

_____

_____

_____

_____

_____

I chuckled over:

_____

_____

_____

_____

_____

I laughed when:

_____

_____

_____

_____

_____

I laughed so hard, I couldn't stop laughing when:

_____

_____

_____

_____

_____

*Optimism is the faith
that leads to achievement.
Nothing can be done without
hope and confidence.*
—Helen Keller

My Private Reflections

In these final pages, capture your learnings, experiences, thoughts, and feelings. Make sure to write down your insights, and identify which practices work best for you. Record how you have or are going to incorporate these activities into your life.

Developing a daily practice is another gift. First, we begin with our commitment to do a particular resiliency-building action every day for thirty days. Choose anything you like to do and do it, even on the hard days. Then notice the progression as the practice moves from something new to something routine. Eventually the routine becomes a habit, and that is when it is harder not to do the practice than to do it. Finally, the routine becomes a daily ritual—and that practice will last you a lifetime.

MY REFLECTIONS

Spend some quiet time just thinking about yourself and capture those mindful thoughts on these pages.

I'm feeling:

_____

_____

_____

_____

_____

I've noticed:

_____

_____

_____

_____

_____

I've been thinking about:

_____

_____

_____

_____

_____

Changes I am considering are:

_____

_____

_____

_____

_____

LOVE LINES TO MYSELF & OTHERS

There is never too much giving and receiving love. Unfortunately, in our busy lives we can forget to tell those we care about just how much they mean to us. These pages have some kind thoughts that you can share. Select five statements every day and express those statements to yourself, your family, and friends.

- I appreciate you.

- I really appreciate all you do for me.

- I appreciate your generosity.

- I appreciate your support.

- I appreciate your kindness.

- I appreciate your patience.

- I appreciate your sense of humor.

- I appreciate your love.

- I love you.

- I admire you.

- I miss you.

- You bring out the best in me.

- You give the best hugs.

- You are my role model.

- You get me.

- You inspire me.

- You are the best.

- You are the light in my life.

- You are amazing.

- You are my rock.

- You are everything to me.

- Thank you for being there for me.

- Thank you for believing in me.

- Thank you for doing everything you do.

- Thank you for caring enough about me to say no.

- Thank you for understanding.

- Thank you for trusting me.

- Thank you being you.

- Thank you for loving me just the way I am.

- Thank you for making me laugh.

LETTER TO MYSELF

These pages are for you to write a letter to yourself to read one year from today. Write from your heart. Write about the special moments that inspired you, the kindnesses you experienced, and your accomplishments from the year. Create the year that you desire as you look forward. Share what you appreciate in your everyday life and acknowledge all the people you love.

Dear Me,

_____

_____

_____

_____

_____

_____

_____

_____

_____

_____

_____

MY PRACTICES

Select the practices you most enjoyed and can envision yourself doing regularly. Check them off and fill in your start date for each practice. Lastly, make note of the time of day and how often you are going to engage with your practices. You can select one practice or many practices—it is your choice.

PRACTICE	START DATE	TIME & FREQUENCY
Daily Gratitude Statements		
Simple Acts of Kindness		
Staying Connected		
The Benefits of Service		
Movement & Exercise		

PRACTICE	START DATE	TIME & FREQUENCY
Being Creative		
Experiencing Quiet Moments		
Practice of Forgiveness		
Reaching for Hard Day Tools		
Writing Your Reflections		

TODAY

Today the pain is less
I breathe deeper and sing louder
Tomorrow may be even better.
I wait with intention and hope,
Knowing always it is possible,
Although others say it is impossible.

I dream to be as I was
Strong, relaxed, boundless energy,
While simultaneously accepting who I am now.
Understanding and receiving all the
gifts the pain brings.
Gratitude, hope, forgiveness,
understanding, compassion,
And most of all being present.

—J. Wilburn

Recommended Reading

Begley, Sharon. *Train Your Mind, Change Your Brain: How a New Science Reveals Our Extraordinary Potential to Transform Ourselves.* New York: Ballantine, 2007.

Emmons, Robert. *Thanks!* New York: Houghton Mifflin Company,

2007. Goleman, Daniel and Richard J. Davidson. *Altered Traits: Science Reveals How Meditation Changes Your Mind, Brain, and Body.* New York: Penguin, 2017.

Hanson, Rick and Forrest Hanson. *Resilient: How to Grow an Unshakable Core of Calm, Strength, and Happiness.* New York: Penguin, 2018.

Hanson, Rick and Richard Mendius. *Buddha's Brain: The Practical Neuroscience of Happiness, Love, and Wisdom.* Oakland, California: New Harbinger, 2009.

Kabat-Zinn, Jon and Richard J. Davidson. *The Mind's Own Physician: A Scientific Dialogue with the Dalai Lama on the Healing Power of Meditation.* Oakland, California: New Harbinger, 2011.

Nerman, Maud. *Healing Pain and Injury.* Richmond, California: Bay Tree, 2013.

Zolli, Andrew and Ann Marie Healy. *Resilience: The Science of Why Things Bounce Back.* New York: Business Plus, 2012.

Acknowledgments

My deepest gratitude to everyone recognized here, who without their support I would never have undertaken this project. First, my family, my family is always first. Thank you for your unshakable belief in my healing, and for believing that I could write these journals even with my health limitations. Knowing you were there for me at every twist and turn made it possible for me to fulfill my dream of sharing this life-altering information with as many people as possible. I am so grateful for you both!

Thank you to all my teachers during this twenty-four-year healing journey. I am truly at a loss for words to describe the depth of my appreciation for you always being there to instruct and assist me. To my yoga teacher, you took me on as a student when I could barely move at times. I will always remember the dignity and respect with which you treat me as I continue to study yoga and work on my recovery. To Pam Lanza & Glenn Hirsch who helped me find, connect, acknowledge, and own both my inner and outer artist when I didn't know I had either. I miss you both, may you rest in peace. To Dr. Maud Nerman for teaching and role modeling that healing is a lifelong journey and to never give up.

I am grateful for my many friends and colleagues who stood with me during these many challenging years, enthusiastically encouraging my writing, art and studies. My dear friend Faith Winthrop who told me this was going to happen. I will celebrate with you in my heart. Aiko Morioka and Cathy River who provided wise, compassionate counsel as I wrote these books. Thank you to Glenn Hartelius, Gordon Sumner, Karen Leveque, Matt Schwartz, John Kirkpatrick, Laurie McFarlane, and Debra Levin for supporting me in so many different ways. I also want to thank the many people around the world who trust me with their joys, fears, accomplishments, hurts, and their hearts. I am honored to be of service to you!

Thank you to those of you who literally these books would not exist without your stellar work. To Luke Schwartz, research assistant extraordinaire for expanding and coordinating my twenty-plus years of research sources. To the amazing team at West Margin Press, I am so grateful to all of you. To Jen Newens, for understanding my vision and providing the platform for this information to reach so many others. To Olivia Ngai for your detailed, precise, and tireless editing. To Rachel Metzger for your thoughtful, innovative designs and your open collaboration. Angie Zbornik for your strategic marketing ideas, innovative execution, and support. I deeply appreciate each and every one of you. Thank you!

About the Author

Janine Wilburn is an award-winning artist, innovator, and writer. She has a master's degree in East West Psychology and is pursuing her PhD. For decades, Janine worked as a marketing professional, receiving recognition for her work with a Cannes Film Festival Bronze Lion, a Clio, and other awards, until a car accident changed her life. Suffering spinal damage, she needed to heal. Through her studies in neuroscience, neuroplasticity, yoga, and meditation, Janine persevered and developed resilience-building practices. The Resiliency Guides are the result of her research, experience, hope, and commitment to help others. Janine lives in San Francisco, California.

I dedicate this book to my amazing son
who inspires me every day with his strength,
compassion, and love in the face of chronic pain.

Text © 2020 by Janine Wilburn

Art Credits: Koru by Kate Bourke from the Noun Project; Flas100/Shutterstock.com; art_of_sun/Shutterstock.com; TairA/Shutterstock.com; photolinc/Shutterstock.com; Podursky/Shutterstock.com; VolodymyrSanych/Shutterstock.com; Khaneeros/Shutterstock.com; Bplanet/Shutterstock.com

ISBN: 9781513264448

Printed in China
1 2 3 4 5

Published by West Margin Press

WEST
MARGIN
PRESS
WestMarginPress.com

Proudly distributed by Ingram Publisher Services

WEST MARGIN PRESS
Publishing Director: Jennifer Newens
Marketing Manager: Angela Zbornik
Editor: Olivia Ngai
Design & Production: Rachel Lopez Metzger